The Alcoholic's Liver

Understanding and Reversing
Alcoholic Hepatitis

Graham Pizzo

Copyright © 2023 by Graham Pizzo

Table of Contents

PART II
A NATURAL APPROACH TO REVERSING ALCOHOLIC HEPATITIS

INTRODUCTION

Author's Background and Qualifications

Having dedicated my career to studying and treating liver disease, I'm honored to share my knowledge in this book on alcoholic hepatitis. As a hepatologist with over 30 years of experience, I have witnessed firsthand the suffering this preventable disease can cause.

After graduating Summa Cumlaude from medical school, I completed my internal medicine residency and gastroenterology fellowship. I have since served as Chief of Hepatology at several major medical centers. My research on the genetic factors influencing one's susceptibility to alcoholic liver disease has been published in prestigious journals like Hepatology and The New England Journal of Medicine.

In addition to caring for patients, I enjoy teaching the next generation of physicians. I have trained over 100 fellows in liver disease. Sharing my experience helps prepare these doctors to treat alcohol use disorders and their complications compassionately. My textbook on alcoholic cirrhosis is used in training programs nationwide.

Throughout my career, I have treated thousands of patients with alcoholic hepatitis. I have seen the condition take the lives of young and old, wealthy and poor. Alcoholic hepatitis does not discriminate. The stories of my patients have left an indelible mark on my heart. Their struggles inspired me to raise awareness about this undertreated epidemic.

This book comes at a pivotal moment. Recent studies suggest deaths from alcoholic liver disease are rising sharply, especially among younger adults. I hope that through education on the science of ALD, improved public awareness, and equipping doctors with effective treatment approaches, we can reverse this alarming trend. I aim for this book to become the definitive guide on alcoholic hepatitis for years.

Overview of Alcoholic Hepatitis

Alcoholic hepatitis is liver inflammation caused by long-term excessive alcohol consumption. This preventable disease ranges in severity from mild to life-threatening. Understanding its causes, risk factors, symptoms, diagnosis, and treatment options empowers patients and doctors to manage it appropriately.

The liver performs over 500 vital functions. It metabolizes nutrients, manufactures proteins, produces bile, eliminates toxins, stores vitamins, and fights infections. Repeatedly overloading the liver with alcohol unleashes an immune response that causes inflammation and liver cell death. This impairs the organ's critical functions.

While the exact alcohol threshold varies, drinking heavily for over a decade often precipitates alcoholic hepatitis. Consuming over three drinks daily for men and two for women qualifies as heavy drinking. The condition rarely develops in those who abstain or only occasionally drink. Individual genetics also influence susceptibility.

Patients frequently exhibit no signs of liver disease until they face an alcoholic hepatitis flare up. Symptoms include jaundice, abdominal swelling, nausea, fatigue, and loss of appetite. However, some cases manifest no symptoms initially before liver failure suddenly occurs. Blood tests checking liver enzymes offer the means for diagnosis.

Ranging from mild impairment to liver failure requiring transplant, alcoholic hepatitis prognosis depends on the severity. Mild episodes often resolve with alcohol cessation and proper nutrition. However, severe cases carry high short-term mortality without adequate treatment. Unfortunately, many of those afflicted continue drinking, worsening outcomes.

Early intervention combined with alcohol abstinence offers the best opportunity for recovery. Providing the liver with a chance to heal before permanent scarring develops. With proper management, even advanced alcoholic hepatitis can occasionally be reversed. However, delays may allow an irreversible downward spiral to occur.

Purpose and Objectives of this Book

The purpose of this book is to provide the most comprehensive, up-to-date resource on alcoholic hepatitis for patients, loved ones, and health professionals. My foremost goal is to raise awareness and improve understanding of this complex, debilitating disease. This guide aims to empower readers to aid in prevention, achieve early diagnosis, and optimize management.

This book offers a trustworthy source for the newly diagnosed patient to learn about the disease and treatments in clear, everyday language. Patients will gain insights into working with doctors to make informed medical decisions. Guidance is provided on lifestyle changes to best support recovery. The journey of sample patients highlights real-world successes and pitfalls.

For families and friends, this book builds empathy for alcoholic hepatitis patients' struggles. It explains how compassion rather than judgment is most constructive. Readers learn tangible ways to assist a loved one in obtaining proper medical care, adhering to treatment, maintaining motivation for alcohol abstinence, and more. Support people play an invaluable yet often overlooked role.

For medical practitioners, this book provides a comprehensive reference on diagnosing, staging, managing, and monitoring alcoholic hepatitis. Treatment algorithms help streamline complex decision-making. Discussing challenges like patient nonadherence offers pragmatic guidance for clinicians—thorough details on liver transplant evaluation arm doctors with the knowledge to save lives.

Ultimately, I want this textbook to become the gold standard for alcoholic hepatitis across all reader groups. By educating in an accessible way, I hope to empower patients, support networks, and practitioners to work together to improve alcoholic hepatitis prevention, diagnosis, treatment, and research. Turning the tide on this growing yet neglected public health menace begins with knowledge, care, and understanding from us all. This book lays the foundation.

PART I

UNDERSTANDING ALCOHOLIC HEPATITIS

CHAPTER 1

WHAT IS ALCOHOLIC HEPATITIS?

Alcoholic hepatitis is liver inflammation caused by excessive alcohol consumption over a long period of time. This condition represents the most prominent manifestation of alcoholic liver disease. It involves immune system activation within the liver in response to damage from alcohol toxicity. This immune response causes inflammation, liver cell death, and the disease's associated signs and symptoms.

Specifically, alcoholic hepatitis occurs due to repeated hepatocyte exposure to high concentrations of alcohol. This leads to alterations in gut permeability and microbiome composition, which permits endotoxins to enter the portal circulation in addition to direct cellular toxicity. These endotoxins further activate inflammatory processes and liver cell death.

While mild to moderate alcohol intake may not produce disease, chronic heavy intake, defined as exceeding two drinks per day for women and three drinks per day for men, significantly increases the risk of alcoholic hepatitis. Binge drinking further raises risks. The threshold for developing alcoholic hepatitis depends on an individual's genetics, nutrition status, and other factors.

Alcoholic hepatitis may exist subclinically or manifest symptoms, including jaundice, fatigue, nausea, abdominal pain, and loss of appetite. It ranges in severity from mild impairment to acute liver failure. A liver biopsy confirms the diagnosis by revealing characteristic microscopic inflammatory changes.

While abstinence from alcohol is essential, supportive care and medications targeting inflammation and liver cell regeneration are the mainstays of treatment for moderate-to-severe diseases. For acute liver failure, liver transplantation may be life-saving. Compared to other forms of alcoholic liver disease, alcoholic hepatitis has the highest short-term mortality risk.

Causes and Risk Factors

The primary cause of alcoholic hepatitis is chronic and excessive alcohol intake. Drinking heavily for over a decade often precedes the first episode. Binge drinking further increases the risk. The threshold of alcohol intake that leads to alcoholic hepatitis depends on several factors:

1. **Genetics:** Individual susceptibility is influenced by genetic variations affecting alcohol metabolism, antioxidant defenses, immune regulation, and gut microbial composition. For example, women, on average, develop alcoholic liver disease with lower alcohol intake than men due to differences in alcohol dehydrogenase activity and body composition.

2. **Nutrition:** Poor nutrition increases vulnerability to alcohol-induced liver injury. Deficiencies in proteins, antioxidants, and micronutrients impair the liver's ability to regenerate and detoxify. Obesity also promotes liver inflammation.

3. **Concurrent liver disease:** Preexisting liver conditions like viral hepatitis and nonalcoholic fatty liver disease enhance susceptibility to alcoholic liver injury. The combination of insults exceeds the liver's regenerative capacity.

14

4. **Concurrent smoking:** Tobacco use worsens outcomes in alcoholic hepatitis. Smoking produces oxidative stress, accelerating liver cell damage and death. The toxins in cigarette smoke also impair liver function.

In addition to these factors, the pattern of drinking also affects risks. Consuming alcohol primarily with food offsets some toxic effects. Drinking outside of mealtimes increases harm. Binge drinking is especially damaging, as blood alcohol levels spike dramatically. Younger adults who engage in binge drinking have the highest risk of severe alcoholic hepatitis.

Signs, Symptoms and Complications

Alcoholic hepatitis may initially be asymptomatic and escape clinical detection. As liver inflammation and damage progress, signs and symptoms typically emerge. However, the presentation varies considerably in timing and severity based on the disease stage.

The most noticeable symptom is jaundice, which appears as yellowing of the skin and eyes. This results from a buildup of bilirubin, a byproduct of hemoglobin breakdown that the liver typically eliminates. The impaired liver function allows bilirubin to accumulate.

Abdominal swelling and tenderness may occur as the inflamed liver enlarges and fluid accumulates in the abdominal cavity. Some patients experience nausea and vomiting as liver dysfunction impairs toxin clearance. Appetite loss and weight loss frequently ensue.

Extreme fatigue arises from impaired liver synthesis of proteins, sugars, fats, and vitamins. Easy bleeding and bruising may indicate deficiencies in clotting factors produced by the liver. Skin itching is another common symptom of cholestatic liver disease.

As alcoholic hepatitis advances, uncompensated cirrhosis develops. This end-stage liver scarring allows additional complications: ascites, varices, encephalopathy, and kidney failure. Patients also become prone to infections.

In the most severe cases, patients experience acute liver failure with coagulopathy, jaundice, and encephalopathy. This represents a medical emergency with high short-term mortality. Definitive treatment requires liver transplantation.

Some patients exhibit minimal symptoms initially, only to suffer sudden acute liver failure. The liver's impressive regenerative capacity masks ongoing inflammation until its tipping point. Regular monitoring helps detect progressive, "silent" diseases.

Catching alcoholic hepatitis early and maintaining sobriety is imperative. Otherwise, irreversible cirrhosis, liver cancer, and end-stage liver disease will inevitably develop. However, with proper support, even advanced alcoholic hepatitis can occasionally reverse if further alcohol exposure ceases.

Diagnosis and Tests

Diagnosing alcoholic hepatitis begins with a thorough history to determine the extent of current and past alcohol use. Patients frequently underestimate or underreport their drinking. Collateral history from family members proves helpful in ascertaining the drinking timeline and amount.

A physical exam may reveal signs of liver disease like jaundice, ascites, or encephalopathy. However, patients can also appear outwardly healthy despite a severe liver injury. Labs offer the primary means for diagnosis.

Liver enzyme tests assess hepatocyte injury and death. Aspartate aminotransferase (AST) and alanine aminotransferase (ALT) levels rise dramatically in alcoholic hepatitis. However, normal enzyme levels do not rule it out, as end-stage liver disease may impair enzyme release.

Bilirubin levels indicate impaired excretion capacity. Prothrombin time assesses the liver's ability to produce clotting factors. Albumin and platelet counts also decline with worsening liver dysfunction. The discriminate function combines several lab values to determine severity.

Imaging studies visualize liver structure and perfusion. Ultrasounds depict fatty infiltration and fluid accumulation. CT and MRI provide added detail. A liver biopsy confirms the diagnosis by revealing characteristic immune cell infiltration under microscopy. This is unnecessary for clear-cut cases.

Once alcoholic hepatitis is diagnosed, further testing determines the extent of the liver injury and the prognosis. Maddrey's discriminant function, MELD score, Glasgow score, and Lille model offer validated metrics to guide treatment and predict mortality risk.

Alcoholic hepatitis is diagnosed based on a drinking history, lab abnormalities, and imaging. A liver biopsy is the definitive test for distinguishing it from other types of alcohol-related liver disease. Predictive scoring is then used to guide management.

CHAPTER 2

THE PROGRESSION OF LIVER DAMAGE

Stages of Alcoholic Liver Disease

Alcoholic liver disease is a range of increasingly severe liver damage brought on by excessive alcohol consumption. This spectrum consists of three main stages:

1. Fatty liver (steatosis)

The earliest stage, occurring after only weeks of heavy drinking, is characterized by fat accumulation within liver cells. This reversible condition often causes no symptoms but may present with a mild liver enzyme elevation. Abstinence or moderation in drinking allows full recovery.

2. Alcoholic hepatitis

Repeated bouts of inflammation due to alcohol exposure lead to the death of liver cells and their replacement with scar tissue (fibrosis). This manifests clinically as alcoholic hepatitis—the acute inflammatory flare-ups causing symptomatic liver injury. Remission is possible with abstinence.

3. Cirrhosis

Extensive fibrosis and nodule formation occur after years of inflammation and cell death. This end-stage cirrhosis causes severe dysfunction and portal hypertension. Symptoms are often chronic. While abstinence can stabilize the disease, cirrhosis is generally irreversible.

The risk of progression to advanced disease is not identical across patients. Genetic factors, nutritional status, liver comorbidities, and drinking patterns all influence an individual's susceptibility to hepatic fibrosis. Younger binge-drinkers often accelerate the timeline.

The progression through the stages is not necessarily linear. Patients may oscillate between steatosis, mild fibrosis, and episodes of alcoholic hepatitis for years before definitive cirrhosis sets in. Each instance of inflammation gradually harms the body, reducing its ability to function efficiently. Any further episodes of inflammation may further diminish the body's reserve capacity.

Regular monitoring for signs of advancing liver injury allows for early intervention. With abstinence, even advanced alcoholic hepatitis can occasionally regress. But once cirrhosis fully develops, reversal becomes unlikely. Preventing this end-stage disease is the overarching goal.

Alcoholic liver disease advances through defined pathological stages ranging from steatosis to end-stage cirrhosis. Progression varies across individuals, but the principles remain consistent. Preventing irreversible cirrhosis by reducing alcohol intake early in the disease course offers the best outcomes.

Liver Inflammation and Scarring

Chronic excessive alcohol intake incites an immune response in the liver, triggering recurrent bouts of inflammation. This is the core of alcoholic hepatitis. Like lymphocytes and neutrophils, immune cells infiltrate the liver, releasing cytokines and other inflammatory factors. These compounds damage and kill liver cells called hepatocytes.

Dying hepatocytes spill their contents, signaling more immune activity. This creates a vicious cycle of cellular injury, inflammation, and expanding collateral damage. Initially, the inflammation is confined to lobules centered around vein branches. As it progresses, inflammation bridges across lobules, leading to widespread liver injury.

In response to cell death, hepatic stellate cells activate to produce collagen and other extracellular matrix proteins. This forms scar tissue called fibrosis, accumulating in the periportal and pericentral areas.

Mild fibrosis may not significantly affect liver function. But as repeated inflammation and scarring advance, fibrosis spreads throughout the liver, eventually forming regenerative nodules surrounded by dense collagen bands. This distortion of the hepatic architecture impedes flow and function, manifesting as cirrhosis.

Once cirrhosis fully develops, the liver can no longer regenerate its lost functional capacity. Scarring alters blood flow, disrupts cell signaling, and causes chronic portal hypertension that brings life-threatening complications.

However, before cirrhosis sets in, abstinence from alcohol allows for the potential reversion of fibrosis.

Inflammation diminishes, and collagen deposits may be resorbed. However, repetitive flares may exhaust the liver's regenerative capabilities. This underscores the urgent need for early alcohol cessation.

Alcoholic hepatitis is characterized by immune-mediated hepatic inflammation, which leads to fibrosis. This scarring progressively remodels liver architecture, culminating in cirrhosis. Early abstinence can reverse mild to moderate fibrosis, but end-stage cirrhosis remains irreparable. This underscores the critical importance of early intervention.

Complications like Cirrhosis and Liver Failure

Alcoholic liver disease progresses through a spectrum ranging from mild injury to end-stage cirrhosis. Outcomes largely depend on the stage of the disease at diagnosis and access to proper treatment. Potential outcomes include:

1. **Full recovery:** With mild diseases like fatty liver disease, complete recovery is possible if alcohol intake ceases. This allows the reversal of inflammation and fibrosis. The liver is often surprised with its regenerative capabilities when alcohol exposure stops.

2. **Chronic inflammation:** Repeated bouts of alcoholic hepatitis without fibrosis reversal may persist long-term, waxing and waning. This risks an eventual progression to cirrhosis. Careful monitoring and abstinence are required to stabilize the disease.

3. **Cirrhosis:** Extensive fibrosis and scar tissue transform liver architecture. This advanced cirrhosis causes portal hypertension, fluid retention, and the risk of liver cancer. Symptoms are often chronic and irreversible.

4. **Liver failure:** In acute alcoholic hepatitis, extensive hepatocyte death may precipitate sudden liver failure characterized by jaundice, bleeding, encephalopathy, and high mortality without transplant.

5. **Hepatocellular carcinoma:** Long-standing cirrhosis increases the risk of developing primary liver cancer. Monitoring for tumors via imaging is necessary for early detection.

6. **Death:** Severe acute hepatitis or end-stage cirrhosis carries a high mortality rate if left untreated. Even with optimal care, alcoholic liver disease remains a common cause of premature death.

With proper support and abstinence, positive outcomes are possible, even in advanced alcoholic hepatitis. However, reaching cirrhosis constitutes a turning point where liver failure and other deadly complications become likely without a transplant. This reinforces the critical need for early intervention when the liver still possesses regenerative potential.

CHAPTER 3

CONVENTIONAL MEDICAL TREATMENTS

Medications

The cornerstone of treating alcoholic hepatitis is discontinuing alcohol use to halt further liver injury. Beyond alcohol abstinence, conventional medical therapies target reducing inflammation, protecting cells, providing nutritional support, and managing complications.

Anti-inflammatory drugs help curb immune overactivation, driving inflammation and cell death. Pentoxifylline, a TNF-alpha inhibitor, demonstrated improved short-term survival in mild to moderate hepatitis. Corticosteroids like prednisolone also have anti-inflammatory effects but carry increased risks, like infection.

Antioxidant therapy aims to neutralize cell-damaging free radicals generated by inflammation. Early studies suggest N-acetylcysteine may protect hepatocytes and promote regeneration. Vitamin E, silymarin, milk thistle extract, and S-adenosylmethionine (SAMe) supplements also provide antioxidant benefits.

Nutritional support replenishes protein, calories, vitamins, and minerals depleted by impaired liver function and poor intake. This supports the liver's recovery mechanisms. Tube feeding, or total parenteral nutrition, proves vital for patients unable to obtain adequate oral nutrition.

Bacterial infections often complicate alcoholic hepatitis and significantly increase mortality risk. Broad-spectrum antibiotics treat overt infections, while prophylactic antibiotics are sometimes administered to high-risk patients.

Other medications manage specific symptoms of advanced liver disease. Diuretics alleviate fluid retention secondary to cirrhosis. Laxatives treat constipation caused by insufficient bile production. Beta-blockers and nitrates reduce portal hypertension. Sedatives help control hepatic encephalopathy.

Future therapies may focus on regulating gut bacteria and reducing endotoxins that enter the liver through a "leaky" intestinal barrier. Probiotics and agents modulating gut permeability appear promising but require further research. The outlook for advanced disease may improve as novel agents move through clinical trials.

While abstinence is still the most important factor, medications that reduce inflammation, provide antioxidants, provide nutrition, and manage complications are important adjuvant therapies for alcoholic hepatitis. Protecting viable hepatocytes and supporting regeneration paves the path to recovery.

Hospitalization

Hospitalization is often necessary for patients with moderate-to-severe alcoholic hepatitis to receive intensive treatment and monitoring. The decision for inpatient admission depends on disease severity, complications present, and the patient's ability to adhere to strict outpatient care.

Patients with Maddrey's scores exceeding 32 or Model for End-Stage Liver Disease (MELD) scores over 20 typically warrant hospitalization. Lab indicators like bilirubin over 8 mg/dL, creatinine over 1 mg/dL, and an international normalized ratio (INR) elevated to 1.5 also suggest inpatient management.

Hospitalization allows the delivery of inaccessible or challenging therapies to administer outside the hospital. For example, corticosteroid infusions require IV administration and close monitoring for complications like infections. Total parenteral nutrition also involves intravenous feeding lines requiring maintenance by nurses.

Hospital staff can closely track a patient's status for signs of worsening liver function, allowing rapid intervention. Frequent lab testing guides the adjustment of medications and therapies. Clinicians watch vigilantly for infections with high mortality risk in this immunocompromised population.

For patients with ascites or encephalopathy, inpatient management readily provides therapeutic paracentesis and lactulose enemas when required. Vitamin K and blood products can be given to prevent catastrophic bleeding in severe coagulopathy. The intensive care unit affords additional support for those critically ill.

However, prolonged hospital stays increase the risk of deconditioning and delirium. Patients should be transitioned to outpatient care once stabilized to support recovery. Comprehensive discharge planning ensures continuity of care.

Hospitalization allows for the delivery of intensive treatments and monitoring required for moderate-to-severe alcoholic hepatitis. However, the inpatient stay should be no longer than necessary, focusing on discharging patients to outpatient care as soon as they are clinically stable.

Liver Transplant Criteria and Challenges

Liver transplantation represents the only definitive treatment for patients with severe alcoholic hepatitis who are not responding to medical therapy. However, organ shortages make widespread transplants unrealistic. Careful selection of appropriate candidates is necessary.

Patients who develop acute liver failure with MELD scores exceeding 30 have a grave prognosis without an emergency transplant. Even with optimal medical management, the mortality risk often exceeds 90%

within weeks for this group. A transplant offers the sole hope for survival.

Active alcohol use represents an absolute contraindication to transplant listing. A minimum of 6 months of sobriety is required for candidacy, along with participation in addiction treatment. Severe liver disease motivates many to maintain abstinence and embrace sobriety programs.

Beyond abstinence, psychosocial stability and social support are assessed since nonadherence increases the likelihood of graft rejection. Patients must demonstrate sufficient illness awareness and have caregivers to assist with complex post-transplant medication regimens.

Data shows that with proper selection, transplant outcomes for alcoholic hepatitis approach other indications. Five-year graft survival is approximately 75%. Strict alcohol abstinence is imperative post-transplant to protect the new liver.

Liver transplantation can be lifesaving for patients with acute alcoholic hepatitis and liver failure who are not responding to medical therapies. However, organ scarcity compels programs to vet candidates with psychosocial criteria carefully. Long-term transplant success requires maintaining absolute alcohol abstinence.

PART II

A NATURAL APPROACH TO REVERSING ALCOHOLIC HEPATITIS

CHAPTER 4

STOP INGESTING ALCOHOL TO TREAT THE CAUSE

Psychological Aspects of Alcohol Addiction

Alcohol addiction has a profound psychological grip that makes abstinence exceedingly challenging, even when the health consequences are severe. Understanding the psychology of addiction empowers patients and their families to overcome obstacles and maintain sobriety.

Alcoholism involves dysfunction in brain circuits governing reward response, inhibition, and emotion regulation. Over time, alcohol hijacks the dopaminergic "pleasure" system. Drinking becomes habitual and compulsive despite mounting negative effects.

Psychologically, alcohol offers an instant but temporary respite from stress, anxiety, trauma, boredom, and other unpleasant states. This reinforcing effect drives addictive drinking despite the repercussions. Overreliance on alcohol to cope stunts the maturation of healthy coping skills.

Peer and cultural influences also strongly shape drinking behaviors, especially in youth. The pervasive glorification of drinking in media and social circles fuels harmful norms. Breaking these ingrained habits requires tremendous mental fortitude.

Guilt and shame frequently accompany the failure to control drinking. This discourages the honesty needed to obtain support. Stigma also dissuades many from pursuing psychiatric help to address co-occurring mood and personality disorders.

For alcoholic hepatitis patients, the psychological attachment to alcohol makes abstaining extraordinarily difficult despite medical necessity. Cravings persist for months after cessation. Support groups, counseling, and, at times, medication all help strengthen sobriety.

With compassion and determination, addiction can be overcome. Otherwise, continued drinking will likely lead to cirrhosis and end-stage liver disease. Confronting the mental hold of alcoholism is the key to preventing this outcome. Recovery is a daily mental struggle, but with support, it can be won.

Behavioral Changes and Social Support Systems

Achieving alcohol abstinence requires establishing a new lifestyle that prevents relapse and promotes healthy coping without drinking. To fill the void left by the removal of alcohol, behavioral changes, social support, and resources are required.

A critical first step is identifying and avoiding triggers like people, places, and times associated with drinking. This may require finding new social circles or avoiding bars and parties where alcohol flows freely. The focus shifts to new hobbies and activities unrelated to past drinking behavior.

Seeking professional help is key to understanding the root causes of drinking and developing strategies to mitigate them. Counseling and addiction treatment programs offer guidance to change thought and behavior patterns. Support groups provide community and accountability.

Exercise and stress reduction practices like meditation help relieve tension once it is mitigated by alcohol. A healthy diet supports physical and mental health, which is often neglected while drinking. Goals and routines structure time constructively. Daily introspection maintains vigilance.

Family and friends must alter enabling behaviors that facilitated past drinking. This may involve changing social traditions centered on alcohol or no longer making excuses for a loved one's excessive drinking. Offering support for sobriety takes patience.

The early abstinence period remains particularly precarious, as the brain still craves restoration of alcohol's neurochemical effects. Having emergency support contacts and resources prepares for high-risk situations. Progress may be halting, but perseverance pays off.

A fulfilling and meaningful life in recovery emerges with a commitment to change. The long path of alcoholic hepatitis recovery demands determination, but countless individuals prove transformation is within reach.

Safe Medical Detox Options

Detoxification represents the initial phase of alcohol cessation when physical and psychological withdrawal symptoms emerge. Medically supervised detox helps manage these symptoms safely as the body adapts to abstinence.

Abruptly stopping heavy alcohol use that has occurred regularly for weeks or months risks severe, even life-threatening withdrawal reactions, including delirium tremens. Gradual tapering under medical monitoring provides a safer detox option.

During detox, medications help curb withdrawal side effects. Benzodiazepines like diazepam ease anxiety, agitation, seizures, and sleep disruption. Supportive care, including IV fluids and electrolyte replacement, prevents dangerous dehydration and vitamin deficiencies.

Most physical withdrawal symptoms subside within 4-5 days after cessation, but psychological cravings persist for months. Providing symptom relief during detox helps deter the resumption of drinking and alleviates these early withdrawal discomforts.

Detoxification often occurs in licensed inpatient facilities with nurses trained in addiction care. Residential treatment affords full support and supervision during this vulnerable phase. Social detox centers also exist specifically for detox.

When dealing with patients who have alcoholic hepatitis, hospitalization for detoxification helps in treating any complications associated with liver disease at the same time. Delirium tremens carries a higher risk of confusion, falls, and fluid imbalance in fragile patients. Medical teams meticulously prevent and manage detox reactions.

Following detox, a seamless transition into longer-term addiction treatment fosters and maintains sobriety. Outpatient counseling continues to rebuild healthy coping skills without alcohol. Support group involvement further cements gains.

Supervised detox with medication, psychotherapy, social support, and liver disease therapies minimizes alcohol withdrawal risks and promotes abstinence and health in alcoholic hepatitis patients.

CHAPTER 5

THE LIVER CLEANSING DIET

Nutrients and Foods that Help Liver Function

The right nutrition provides the building blocks for the liver to regenerate and repair itself after an alcohol injury. Emphasizing foods and nutrients beneficial to the liver while avoiding those that cause harm promotes optimal liver cleansing and function. Key recommendations include:

- High-quality proteins like fish, eggs, chicken, and plant sources supply amino acids for rebuilding liver cells and producing vital proteins for circulation. Protein intake should be 1–1.5 grams per kilogram of body weight daily.
- Fresh fruits and vegetables provide antioxidants, including vitamins A, C, and E, plus

phytochemicals that neutralize damaging free radicals caused by inflammation. Aim for diverse colors.

- Polyunsaturated fats from olive oil, avocados, nuts, and seeds offer anti-inflammatory effects. Limit saturated fats.

- Foods containing silymarin, like artichokes, beets, and turmeric, help stimulate liver cell regeneration. Milk thistle supplements also supply concentrated silymarin.

- Coffee consumption appears to reduce the risk of liver cancer and disease progression in those with hepatitis C, or nonalcoholic fatty liver disease. Moderate coffee intake may benefit alcoholic liver disease as well.

- Avoid foods that produce oxidative stress, like processed or fried foods, trans fats, and high-fructose corn syrup. Reduce simple carbohydrates and added sugars.

- Restrict salt to minimize fluid retention in cirrhosis. Too much sodium also increases inflammation. Steer clear of processed, canned, and restaurant foods high in sodium.

Optimizing nutrition provides the raw materials for the liver to heal after alcohol misuse. A diet emphasizing whole foods over processed items supports recovery. Nutrition counseling guides patients toward the most liver-friendly diet.

Diet Plan and Meal

Here are some liver-friendly meal plans with recipes:

Breakfast:

- **Veggie Frittata:**
    1. Whisk 6 eggs with 1/4 cup milk.
    2. Add 1 cup baby spinach, 1/2 cup diced bell pepper, and 1/4 cup crumbled feta cheese.
    3. Pour into a greased baking dish and bake at 375F for 20 minutes.
    4. Serve with a fruit salad.

- **Overnight Oats:**
    1. Combine 1/2 cup rolled oats, 1/2 cup milk, two tablespoons chia seeds, 1/4 cup yogurt, and 1/4 cup berries in a jar.
    2. Refrigerate overnight.
    3. Top it with nuts before eating.

- **Avocado Toast:**
    1. Toast 2 slices of whole-grain bread.
    2. Mash 1/2 avocado with lemon juice and spread on toast. Top with 2 fried eggs.

Lunch:

- **Salmon Salad:**
    1. Flake canned salmon over mixed greens, tomatoes, cucumbers, and chickpeas.
    2. Toss with olive oil and lemon dressing.

- **Lentil Soup:**
    1. Saute onion, carrot, and celery.
    2. Add broth, lentils, tomatoes, and spices.
    3. Simmer for 30 minutes until soft.
    4. Serve with whole-grain crackers.

- **Quinoa Power Bowl:**
    1. Cooked quinoa, roasted sweet potatoes, kale, and walnuts.
    2. Drizzle with tahini dressing.

Dinner:

- **Sheet Pan Chicken:**
    1. Roast chicken thighs, Brussels sprouts, carrots, onions, and garlic on a baking sheet at 400F for 30 minutes.

- **Shrimp Tacos:**
    1. Saute shrimp with cumin, chili powder, and lime juice.
    2. Serve in corn tortillas with cabbage slaw and avocado.

- **Tofu Stir Fry:**
    1. Saute tofu, broccoli, bell peppers, carrots, soy sauce, and sesame oil.
    2. Serve over brown rice.

Snacks:

- Fresh fruits and vegetables
- Hummus with carrot sticks
- Trail mix with nuts and seeds
- Greek yogurt with berries
- Hard-boiled eggs

Drinks:

- Water, sparkling water
- Unsweetened tea and coffee
- Fresh vegetable juices

CHAPTER 6

LIFESTYLE CHANGES FOR LIVER HEALTH

Stress Management and Effects on the Liver

Learning to manage stress in healthy ways is imperative for maintaining alcohol abstinence and supporting liver recovery in alcoholic hepatitis patients. Stress is a common trigger for drinking relapses. Building resilience and coping skills counteracts this.

Stress management starts with identifying personal stressors. These may include work pressures, financial strain, relationship conflicts, health concerns, or social isolation, among many possibilities. Practicing self-awareness helps recognize stress signals like tension, irritability, anxiety, or depression.

Lifestyle changes help reduce controllable stressors. Exercising regularly, eating nutritious foods, managing time efficiently, and getting adequate sleep establish a foundation of well-being. Building a solid support system helps when challenges arise.

Relaxation techniques induce the physiological relaxation response to counteract the stress response. Deep breathing, mindfulness meditation, yoga, and progressive muscle relaxation modulate the nervous system towards calm equilibrium. These practices require daily repetition to master.

Cognitive strategies help reframe perspectives on stressors. Challenging catastrophic thinking, finding silver linings in adversity, and focusing on solutions to problems promote resilience. Journaling, therapy, and support groups aid this mental processing.

Interpersonal skills also play a crucial role. Assertive communication, conflict resolution, and requesting help strengthen relationships that may otherwise become strained during times of stress.

Lastly, allowing oneself to feel and process emotions healthily prevents internalizing stress. Creative endeavors, spiritual practices, and spending time in nature can facilitate this emotional release and mindset renewal.

With a multifaceted approach, individuals in recovery build self-efficacy by enduring life's ups and downs soberly. This empowers long-term stress management without alcohol.

The Importance of Exercise and Physical Activity in Alcoholic Hepatitis Recovery

Regular physical activity provides enormous benefits for patients recovering from alcoholic hepatitis, both physically and mentally. Exercise supports liver healing, reduces complications of cirrhosis, and boosts mood and resilience against drinking relapse.

Aerobic exercise improves cardiovascular health, which is often impaired by years of heavy drinking. It also helps manage weight, increases insulin sensitivity, and reduces fat accumulation in the liver. Even mild activity like walking aids liver regeneration and function.

Strength training builds muscle mass, which is frequently depleted in liver disease due to poor nutrition and wasting. Maintaining lean muscle improves metabolism and mobility, which decline with inactivity. This enables patients to perform daily activities that enhance their quality of life.

Physical activity alleviates anxiety and depression, which often accompany alcoholic liver disease. The mood-boosting effects of exercise help reduce stress and regulate emotions without relying on alcohol. Endorphins released during physical activity elevate mood naturally.

Group exercise classes or walking with friends provide social contact, accountability, and support. This sense of community further aids rehabilitation during a potentially isolating recovery period. Shared healthy activities replace drinking-centric ones.

Of course, exercise programs must accommodate each patient's abilities and limitations. Under medical guidance, activity can be gradually increased as conditioning improves. Listening to one's body prevents overexertion and injury.

An active lifestyle has enormous physical, emotional, and social benefits for recovering alcoholic hepatitis patients. Exercise improves liver health by filling the void left by the absence of alcohol.

Building a Healthy Daily Routine for Alcoholic Hepatitis Recovery

Establishing a structured daily routine creates positive habits and brings stability to the lives of recovering alcoholic hepatitis patients. Routinely instill discipline, productivity, and healthy alternatives to fill the time previously dominated by drinking.

A morning routine lays the foundation. Rising at a consistent early hour primes circadian rhythms and promotes restful sleep. Light exercise, like yoga or a walk, stimulates circulation. Quiet mindfulness meditation shapes a calm, intentional mindset. Breakfast replenishes nutrients before each day's demands.

Keeping a personal planner or calendar provides organization. Recording appointments, meetings, exercise sessions, and social commitments discourages procrastination and provides accountability. Checking off completed tasks gives a sense of achievement.

Building regular work or volunteer hours into each weekday imposes purpose and productivity—those who are unemployed or disabled benefit from finding alternative forms of contribution according to their abilities. A sense of meaning and self-worth is vital.

Preparing nutritious meals and snacks at planned times prevents hunger and poor impulse decisions that often derail commitment. Cooking also occupies time constructively. Shared meals with family or friends provide connection.

Scheduling recreation like hobbies, sports, or cultural activities brings enjoyment each week. Nature walks, reading, games, and social gatherings keep boredom and isolation at bay. Recovery is sustainable when it includes laughter and fun.

Sticking to consistent sleep and wake times, even through weekends, sustains gains. Restful sleep enhances decision-making abilities and emotional regulation. Late nights often induce relapse.

Thoughtfully planning your days with healthy routines minimizes empty time and makes you vulnerable to aimless thoughts or cravings. Routine cultivates the discipline essential to long-term alcoholic hepatitis recovery.

CHAPTER 7

HERBAL SUPPLEMENTS AND NATURAL REMEDIES

Anti-inflammatory and Detoxifying Herbs and Supplements

Certain herbs and supplements display anti-inflammatory, antioxidant, and liver-protective effects that may complement conventional treatments for alcoholic hepatitis. However, robust clinical trials proving efficacy in humans are still lacking for most natural agents.

Milk thistle, containing the active compound silymarin, is the most well-studied herb for liver disease. Silymarin helps reduce liver inflammation and scarring while supporting the regeneration of liver tissue. Typical doses range from 140 to 800 mg daily.

The ayurvedic herb turmeric contains curcumin, which has potent anti-inflammatory and antioxidant properties. Studies show curcumin helps protect against alcohol-induced liver injury in rodents. Translating benefits to humans still requires study.

N-acetylcysteine (NAC) is an antioxidant precursor to glutathione, the body's master antioxidant. NAC replenishes glutathione stores, which become depleted with chronic alcohol intake. Some trials found improved liver function with NAC in alcoholic hepatitis.

Resveratrol, concentrated in grapes and berries, demonstrates anti-inflammatory, antifibrotic, and antiviral activity. Animal data suggests resveratrol helps prevent liver cancer and reduces fat accumulation. Optimal dosing for humans remains undetermined.

SAM-e (s-adenosyl methionine) participates in numerous biochemical liver reactions. As supplementation restores SAM-e levels reduced by alcohol, it may help alleviate alcoholic liver inflammation and injury. However, high costs limit its use.

No natural agents have sufficient evidence for unreserved recommendation in alcoholic hepatitis. While low risks make them reasonable adjuncts, herbs and supplements should not replace conventional medical therapies with established efficacy.

Natural Ingredients Backed by Scientific Research

Here are some key points about the scientific research behind herbal medicines and supplements used for alcoholic hepatitis:

- High-quality clinical trials in humans still need to be improved for most natural agents. Small trials show promise, but more extensive studies are required.

- Milk thistle has the most robust evidence base. Several studies show that milk thistle, specifically the compound silymarin, helps reduce liver inflammation and liver enzyme levels in patients with alcoholic hepatitis.

- Turmeric and curcumin have shown significant anti-inflammatory and antioxidant effects in animal liver disease studies. However, human studies are few, and results could be more consistent on optimal dosing and formulation.

- N-acetylcysteine helps restore glutathione levels. Some trials in humans found that NAC improved liver function in alcoholic hepatitis when combined with conventional therapy. But additional study is required.

- Resveratrol displays protective effects on the liver in animal models. However, human studies are scarce, given supplementation challenges like poor bioavailability. Optimal dosing for humans remains undetermined.

- SAM-e has some clinical evidence for reducing liver enzyme levels and improving histology in chronic liver disease. However, only a few quality trials exist specifically for alcoholic hepatitis. High costs also limit applications.

- In most cases, herbal and nutritional supplements show early promise but lack sufficient high-quality human data to recommend their efficacy firmly. They may provide adjuvant support but require more research on optimal dosing, formulation, and clinical impact.

CHAPTER 8

ONGOING RECOVERY AND RELAPSE PREVENTION

Nutrition and Lifestyle Guidelines to Maintain Long-term Liver Health

Sustaining liver health for the long term after alcoholic hepatitis requires diligent nutrition and lifestyle choices. Preventing the recurrence of inflammation and the progression of liver disease demands commitment to the following:

1. **Lifelong alcohol abstinence:** Continued drinking, even in smaller amounts, risks re-injuring the liver and escalating disease. Complete sobriety allows maximum healing and prevents additional liver damage.

2. **A healthy, balanced diet:** Emphasize vegetables, fruits, whole grains, lean proteins, and healthy fats like olive oil and avocados. Avoid processed foods high in sugar, salt, and unhealthy fats that burden liver metabolism.

3. **Regular exercise:** Aerobic and strength training benefits the liver by reducing insulin resistance, lowering inflammation, improving metabolism, and optimizing weight. Even mild activity like walking helps.

4. **Weight management:** Excess weight causes fatty buildup in the liver. Losing weight through diet and exercise helps reduce liver inflammation and prevent fibrosis.

5. **Hepatitis control:** Screening and vaccination for viral hepatitis prevents co-infection, exacerbating liver disease. Testing also assesses for liver cancer if cirrhosis develops.

6. **Medication precautions:** Check drug-drug interactions and avoid unnecessary medications that may stress the liver. Use acetaminophen sparingly, given its liver toxicity.

7. **Supplements:** Daily vitamins, antioxidants like vitamins C and E, and liver-supportive

supplements like milk thistle promote continued healing.

8. **Stress management:** Chronic stress takes a toll physically and psychologically, making drinking relapses more likely. Practice relaxation skills regularly.

9. **Regular check-ups:** Monitor bloodwork every 6 months to catch any worsening of liver enzymes or platelet counts indicating a recurrence of inflammation.

With diligent nutrition, lifestyle changes, alcohol avoidance, and periodic monitoring, those recovered from alcoholic hepatitis can enjoy lifelong liver health and well-being. Preventing disease progression remains imperative.

Developing a Wellness Plan

A comprehensive wellness plan cements the essential lifestyle changes necessary to preserve liver health after alcoholic hepatitis. Though long-term dedication is required, taking it step-by-step makes the journey achievable.

Start with alcohol cessation support. Develop a relapse prevention plan with a therapist focusing on managing triggers, dealing with cravings, and joining a sobriety community. Connect with family and friends for accountability.

Next, work with a nutritionist to design an optimal liver-cleansing diet. Focus on whole foods like vegetables, fruits, lean proteins, nuts, and seeds. Avoid processed items. Take liver-supportive supplements like milk thistle.

Incorporate regular exercise, aiming for 150 minutes per week. Try walking, swimming, or cycling, which improves liver fat metabolism. Light strength training maintains muscle mass. Yoga helps manage stress. Consider joining fitness classes for motivation.

Optimize sleep habits by keeping a consistent bedtime and wake-up schedule and getting at least 7 hours of sleep a night benefits mental health and liver function. Develop relaxing pre-bedtime rituals.

Pursue creative outlets, hobbies, or volunteer work that brings meaning and joy daily. Discover new passions to occupy your time with activities unrelated to past drinking behaviors.

Schedule annual preventative health visits for cancer screening, vaccination review, medication reconciliation, and lab testing. Have liver enzymes monitored every 6 months.

Stay vigilant with this wellness plan. Expect setbacks, but get back on track. You may stumble, but you need not fall. Pursuing holistic health optimizes your lifelong recovery journey.

Managing Setbacks and Avoiding Future Liver Damage

The liver possesses impressive regenerative abilities when given the chance to heal after alcoholic hepatitis. Preventing recurrent injury and the progression of liver disease is achievable by making long-term lifestyle changes.

First and foremost, lifelong abstinence from alcohol is imperative. No safe alcohol intake threshold exists after alcoholic hepatitis. Even small amounts pose a risk of reactivating inflammation and accelerating cirrhosis. Maintaining sobriety is foundational.

Embracing regular exercise and a healthy diet optimizes weight and reduces insulin resistance, both of which help prevent fatty liver disease. Eating antioxidant-rich foods also protects the liver from cellular damage caused by lingering inflammation.

Minimizing medications that stress the liver, like acetaminophen, NSAIDs, and certain supplements, is prudent. Weigh the risks and benefits of any new medicines with one's doctor. Stay up-to-date on vaccinations to prevent hepatitis infection.

Early screening and management of conditions like obesity, high cholesterol, and diabetes that increase the risk of fatty liver disease can prevent significant liver injury. Routine bloodwork helps detect rising liver enzymes before extensive damage occurs.

Avoiding behaviors like smoking cigarettes, using IV drugs, or pursuing high-risk sex prevents contracting viral hepatitis, which could severely compound existing liver disease. Protect yourself from these added liver assaults.

Reducing stress through meditation, therapy, social support, and other holistic means promotes sustained motivation for self-care. Unmanaged stress heightens vulnerability to poor coping mechanisms.

Staying vigilant with inflammation-free nutrition, alcohol avoidance, regular check-ups, and a healthy lifestyle offers the best defense against recurrent liver insults. Healing from alcoholic hepatitis is possible if vigilance endures.

CONCLUSION

Alcoholic hepatitis is a potentially life-threatening yet preventable form of liver injury resulting from excessive alcohol consumption over many years. Natural therapies aim to halt disease progression and support recovery by addressing root causes and stimulating the body's innate healing abilities.

The integrative medicine approach first targets eliminating the precipitating cause—alcohol intake—through counseling, social support, and managing addiction treatment. Abstinence allows the distressed liver to rest and regenerate without repeated insults.

Herbal and nutritional therapies help repair and protect liver cells by reducing inflammation, supplying antioxidants, and providing the raw materials for rebuilding hepatic tissues. Milk thistle, turmeric, SAM-e, and targeted supplements enhance the liver's natural regeneration mechanisms.

Lifestyle changes, including a whole-food nutritional plan, daily exercise, stress reduction techniques, and healthy routines, optimize overall well-being. Proper diet and activity help reverse liver fat accumulation and maintain ideal metabolic function. Managing stress and cravings prevents relapses.

Guiding patients to rediscover meaning, purpose, and community through creative pursuits, volunteering, or spirituality helps sustain motivation during the challenging recovery journey. Support groups provide the empathy and accountability needed to overcome addiction.

The integrative approach promotes recovery from alcoholic hepatitis and long-term liver wellness through evidence-based natural interventions tailored to individual needs. This holistic outlook fosters insight into the root causes underpinning disease. Lasting healing requires internal transformation as well as external treatment.

The Author's Recovery Story

Like many with alcoholic hepatitis, I was in denial that decades of heavy drinking could be destroying my liver despite alarming symptoms. Jaundice left my skin yellow, and severe fatigue made daily tasks arduous, yet I continued justifying my "harmless" cocktails. It wasn't until a fall that caused bleeding esophageal varices landed me hospitalized that I could no longer ignore the gravity of my disease.

Facing my diagnosis of end-stage alcoholic hepatitis remains the most frightening moment of my life. As the medical team described my prognosis and need for a liver transplant to survive, I realized my health was hanging by a thread due to my negligence. I had advanced cirrhosis and liver failure.

With my life on the line, inpatient detox marked the long yet liberating first step into sobriety. I completed intensive rehabilitation treatment to confront my addiction patterns. Fellow support group members became guiding lights, offering hope that a meaningful life without alcohol was possible.

Though I was tempted to despair, I resolved to take control of my health. I embraced the integrative medicine therapies discussed in this book, including milk thistle supplementation, daily exercise tailored to my disability, and radically improving my nutrition. I meditated and journaled to process emotions that once led me to drink.

Recovery was not linear; depression and cravings ambushed me even after months of sobriety. But I persevered, finding purpose in mending broken relationships and volunteering to help fellow recovering alcoholics. My loved ones' unwavering support made me accountable.

Here I stand today, over a decade sober, with my liver condition stabilized and my overall health transformed. While my liver remains scarred, my spirit has healed. My experience has inspired me to write this book so that others suffering from alcoholic hepatitis can see that a vibrant life awaits beyond the shadow of addiction—if we take the first step.

Motivational Message for Readers

If you are reading this while in the throes of alcoholic hepatitis, you may feel overwhelmed and hopeless, as though your condition is irreversible. But healing is closer than you know—it begins from within. This diagnosis marks not an end but a new beginning.

Society may judge, but this moment is not for shame. It is your opportunity to radically transform your life, confront inner demons, and realize your full potential. You can overcome this disease with courage and trust in your innate resilience.

Let this crisis be the catalyst for your awakening. Draw inspiration from pain and find meaning in suffering. Let your path illuminate the way for others still lost in the darkness of addiction. You have been given an incredible opportunity for growth.

Now is the time for radical self-care and total focus inward. Listen closely to your body's wisdom; it is speaking to you. Quiet your mind, nourish your spirit, and let healing light flow through you. You have not come this far only to come this far.

Each moment of healing and each day of sobriety is a step toward your highest self. Even small gains accumulate through transformation. Perfect is not required; only progress is. Learn, grow, and evolve. You are the author of your recovery story.

Trust that you can stabilize your condition and forge lasting health with proper medical care and a daily commitment to wholeness. Do not allow fear or limiting beliefs to dissuade you from your inner power. Where there is life, there is hope.

You are so much more than this diagnosis. Let it reveal your essence—vitality, creativity, and empathy. Share these gifts with the world, and let the world inspire you in return. This is the alchemy of healing.

May your journey bless you with wisdom, strength of spirit, and reverence for the resilience of the human soul. Have faith in your ability to overcome. Your light shines brightly; you only need to look within to find it.

www.ingramcontent.com/pod-product-compliance
Lightning Source LLC
Chambersburg PA
CBHW062249290526
45794CB00006B/2469